Keto Diet Cookies Recipes for Beginners

Enjoy this Collection of Cookies and Lose Weight, Boost your Metabolism and your Health

Jessica Simpson

Contents

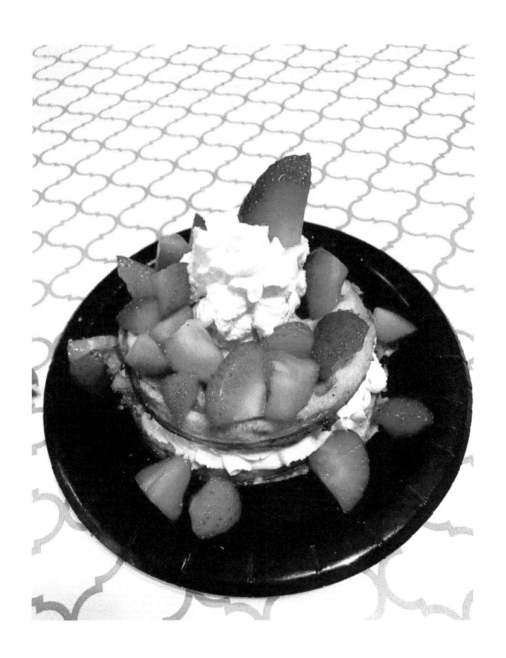

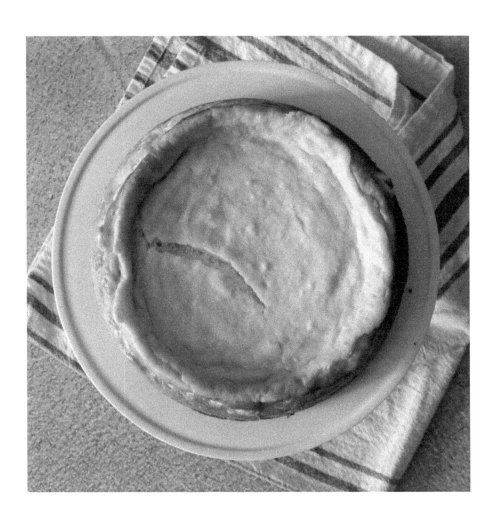

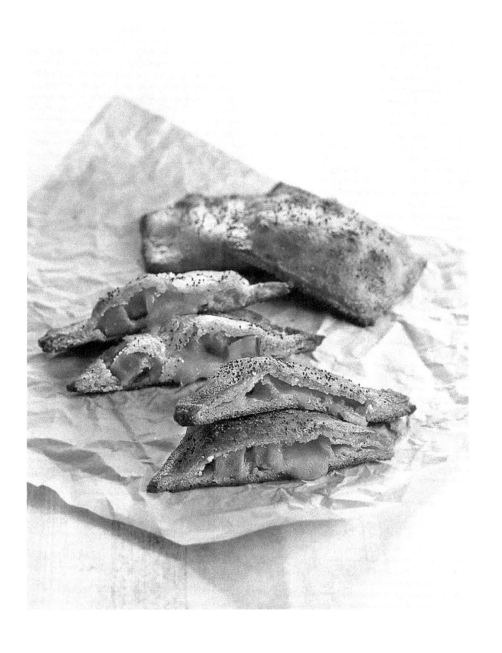

Snickerdoodles

Servings: 12

Cooking Time: 15 Minutes

Ingredients:

- For the Cookies:
- 2 cups superfine almond flour
- ½ cup salted butter, softened
- Pinch of kosher salt
- ¾ cup erythritol granulated sweetener
- ½ tsp baking soda
- For the Coating:
- 2 tbsp erythritol granulated sweetener
- 1 tsp ground cinnamon

Directions:

1. Preheat your oven to 350 degrees F.
2. Whisk all the cookie ingredients in a medium-sized bowl.
3. Make 16 small balls out of this mixture and place them on a baking sheet lined with wax paper.
4. Mix cinnamon with sweetener in a shallow dish and sprinkle this mixture over the balls.
5. Flatten the balls lightly then bake them for 1minutes.
6. Serve.

Nutrition Info: Calories 198 Total Fat 19.2 g Saturated Fat 11.5 g Cholesterol 123 mg Sodium 142 mg Total Carbs 4.5 g Sugar 3.3 g Fiber 0.3 g Protein 3.4 g

Chocolate Cookies

Servings: 20

Cooking Time: 55 Minutes

Ingredients:

- 3/4 cup coconut flour
- 1/2 cup monk fruit sweetener
- 2 cups Nutella, low-carb

Directions:

1. Place all the ingredients in a large bowl and stir well until thick batter comes together.
2. Shape the mixture into cookie balls and place on a baking tray lined with parchment paper.
3. Place the baking tray into the refrigerator and chill for 45 minutes or until firm. Serve straightaway.

Nutrition Info: Calories: 98 Cal, Carbs: 5 g, Fat: 8 g, Protein: g, Fiber: 3 g.

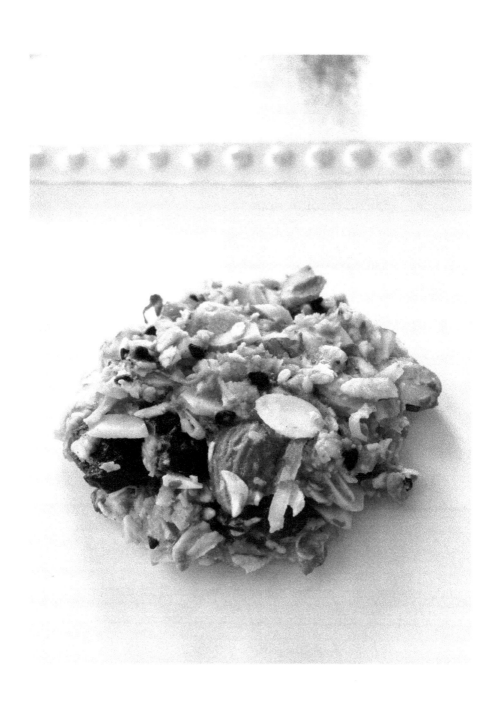

Coconut Vanilla Cookies

Servings: 4

Cooking Time: 10 Minutes

Ingredients:

- 6 tablespoons coconut flour
- ¾ teaspoon baking powder
- 1/8 teaspoon salt
- 3 tablespoons butter
- 1/6 cup coconut oil
- 6 tablespoons swerve
- 2 large eggs
- 1/2 tablespoon coconut milk
- 1/2 teaspoon vanilla essence

Directions:

1. Let your oven preheat at 375 degrees F.
2. Line a baking sheet with wax paper.
3. Beat all the wet ingredients in a food processor.
4. Stir in rest of the ingredients and mix well.
5. Divide the dough into small cookies on the cookie sheet.
6. Bake for 10 mins in the preheated oven.
7. Allow the cookies to cool in 15 minutes.
8. Serve.

Nutrition Info: Calories 151 ;Total Fat 14.7 g ;Saturated Fat 1.5 g ;Cholesterol 13 mg ;Sodium 53 mg ;Total Carbs 1.5 g ;Sugar 0.3 g ;Fiber 0.1 g ;Protein 0.8 g

Keto Blueberry Muffins

Servings: 12

Cooking Time: 25 Minutes

Ingredients:

- 2 and ½ cups of blanched almond flour
- ½ Cup of Erythritol
- 1 and ½ teaspoons of Gluten-free baking powder
- ¼ Teaspoon of Sea salt
- 1/3 Cup of Coconut oil
- 1/3 Cup of Unsweetened almond milk
- 3 large Eggs
- ½ Teaspoon of Vanilla extract
- ¾ Cup of Blueberries

Directions:

1. Preheat your oven to a temperature of about 350 F.
2. Line a standard muffin tray with 1parchment muffin liners.
3. In a large bowl, stir all together the erythritol with the baking powder and the sea salt.
4. Mix in the coconut oil; the almond milk, the eggs and the vanilla extract.
5. Add in the blueberries; then equally distribute the batter among the muffin cups.
6. Bake your muffins for about 20 to 25 minutes.

7. Serve and enjoy your sumptuous muffins!

Nutrition Info: Calories: 217;Fat: 19 g;Carbohydrates: 6g;Fiber: 3g;Protein: 8

Easy Coconut Cookies

Servings: 40

Cooking Time: 10 Minutes

Ingredients:

- 4 cups unsweetened shredded coconut
- 12 cup unsweetened coconut milk
- 14 cup erythritol
- 14 tsp vanilla

Directions:

1. Add all ingredients to the food processor and process until sticky.
2. Transfer mixture to the large bowl.
3. Make a small ball from mixture and place on a plate.
4. Press each ball lightly into a cookie shape and place in the fridge until firm.
5. Serve and enjoy.

Nutrition Info: Per Servings: Net Carbs: 0.9g; Calories: 79; Total Fat: 7.1g; Saturated Fat: 2g Protein: 0.9g; Carbs: 2.6g; Fiber: 1.7g; Sugar: 0.9g; Fat 86% Protein 7% Carbs 7%

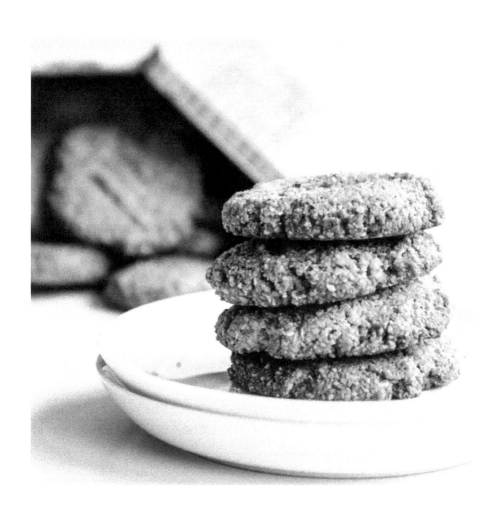

Hazelnut, Coconut And Orange Cookies

Servings: 16

Cooking Time:30 Minutes

Ingredients:

- 1 cup ground almonds
- 2 cups unsweetened coconut thread
- 1 cup chopped hazelnuts
- 1 tsp Stevia/your preferred keto sweetener
- Pinch of salt
- 1 tsp baking powder
- 4 oz butter, melted
- 2 eggs
- Juice and zest of 1 orange

Directions:

1. Preheat the oven to 360 degrees Fahrenheit and line a baking tray with baking paper
2. Combine the ground almonds, coconut thread, hazelnuts, sweetener, salt and baking powder in a large bowl
3. In a separate bowl, whisk together the melted butter, eggs, orange juice and zest
4. Pour the wet ingredients into the dry ingredients and stir to combine

5. Place dollops of batter onto your prepared baking tray. Don't worry if the batter dollops look a little messy, they're meant to be!
6. Place the tray into the preheated oven and bake for about 20 minutes or until the cookies are golden brown
7. Leave the cookies to cool completely before eating!

Nutrition Info: Calories: 192;Fat: 19 grams ;Protein: 4 grams ;Total carbs: 5 grams ;Net carbs: 3 grams

Chocolate Chip Cookies

Servings: 20

Cooking Time:25 Minutes

Ingredients:

- 2 tsp vanilla extract
- 5 oz butter, melted
- 2 eggs
- 2 cups ground almonds
- 1 ½ tsp Stevia/your preferred keto sweetener
- 6 oz 72% cocoa dark chocolate, roughly chopped
- 2 tsp baking powder
- Pinch of salt

Directions:

1. Preheat the oven to 360 degrees Fahrenheit and line a baking tray with baking paper
2. In a large bowl, whisk together the vanilla, melted butter and eggs
3. Stir the ground almonds, sweetener, chocolate, baking powder and salt into the egg/butter mixture until thoroughly combined
4. Roll the dough into 20 balls and place them onto your prepared tray

5. Use a fork to press down the cookie dough balls and place the tray into the oven to bake for about 1minutes or until the cookies are just turning golden but still soft
6. Leave the cookies to cool before eating or storing away in an airtight container

Nutrition Info: Calories: 163;Fat: 15 grams ;Protein: 3 grams ;Total carbs: 4 grams ;Net carbs: 2 grams

Pecan Shortbread Cookies

Servings: 6

Cooking Time: 15 Minutes

Ingredients:

- ¾ cup almond flour
- ¼ cup coconut flour
- 1 large egg
- 4 tbsp butter, melted
- ½ cup erythritol
- 1 tsp vanilla extract
- ½ tsp baking powder
- ¼ tsp xanthan gum
- 1/3 cup raw pecans, crushed

Directions:

1. Add all dry ingredients to a bowl then mix well with a fork.
2. Whisk melted butter and vanilla extract in a separate bowl then stir in half of the dry mixture.
3. Add egg and mix well until combined. Now, stir in the remaining dry mixture.
4. Mix this well until fully incorporated.
5. Add pecans to the cookie dough and mix well.
6. Place the dough on wax paper and form it into a rectangular log with your hands.

7. Cover it with more wax paper and freeze for 30 minutes.

8. Meanwhile, preheat your oven for 5 minutes at 350 degrees F.

9. Layer a cookie sheet with wax paper and set it aside.

10. Slice the dough log into ¼-inch thick slices.

11. Place the slices on the cookie sheet and bake them for 15 minutes.

12. Allow them to cool then serve.

Nutrition Info: Calories 121 Total Fat 12.9 g Saturated Fat 5.1 g Cholesterol 17 mg Sodium 28 mg Total Carbs 8.1 g Sugar 1.8 g Fiber 0.4 g Protein 5.4 g

Keto Snickerdoodle Cookies

Servings: 8

Cooking Time: 12 Minutes

Ingredients:

- For cookies (wet ingredients):
- 1 egg
- ½ cup almond butter
- 2 tablespoons solid coconut oil, at room temperature
- 1 teaspoon vanilla extract
- ¼ cup almond butter
- For cookies (dry ingredients)
- ¾ cup + 2 tablespoons almond flour
- ½ teaspoon baking soda
- A pinch pink Himalayan salt
- ½ cup coconut flour
- 1 teaspoon cream of tartar
- ½ teaspoon ground cinnamon
- ¾ cup monk fruit sweetener
- For coating:
- ½ tablespoon ground cinnamon
- 1 ½ tablespoons monk fruit sweetener

Directions:

1. Add all the dry ingredients into a bowl and stir.

2. Add all the wet ingredients into another bowl. Whisk with an electric hand mixer until ingredients are well combined.

3. Add dry ingredients into the bowl of wet ingredients, a little at a time and mix well by hand each time, until well combined.

4. Chill the dough for 15 minutes.

5. Divide the dough into 8 equal portions and shape into balls. Place on a plate.

6. Mix cinnamon and sweetener together in a medium bowl

7. Dredge the balls in the cinnamon mixture.

8. Line a baking sheet with parchment paper. Place the balls on the baking sheet. Leave sufficient gap between the cookies.

9. Press the cookies with the back of a glass and flatten them.

10. Bake in a preheated oven at 350° F for about – 13 minutes or until light golden brown. Bake in batches.

11. Remove the baking sheet from the oven and let cookies cool on the baking sheet completely.

12. Transfer into an airtight container. These can keep for 7 – 8 days in the refrigerator. If you freeze the cookies they can keep for 3 months.

Nutrition Info: per Servings: Calories: 281.9 kcal, Fat: 23.9 g, Carbohydrates: 11.9 g, Protein: 9.6 g

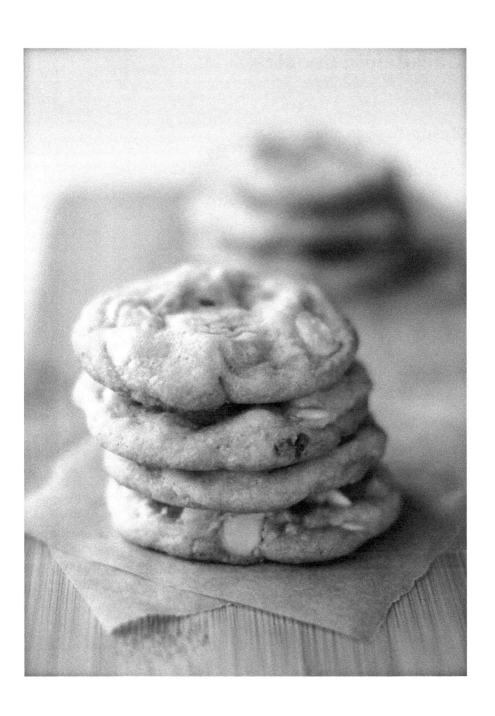

Macadamia Cookies

Servings: 11

Cooking Time: 10 Minutes

Ingredients:

- 1/2 cup coconut oil, melted
- 2 tablespoons almond butter
- 1 egg
- 1 1/2 cup almond flour
- 2 tablespoons unsweetened cocoa powder
- 1/2 cup granulated erythritol sweetener
- 1 teaspoon vanilla extract
- 1/2 teaspoon baking soda
- 1/4 cup chopped macadamia nuts
- 1 Pinch of salt

Directions:

1. Start by preheating your oven to a temperature of about 350 F.
2. Combine the almond butter with the coconut oil, the almond flour, the cocoa powder, the swerve, the vanilla extract, the baking soda, the chopped macadamia nut and the salt in a large mixing bowl.
3. Mix your ingredients very well with a fork or a spoon; then set it aside.

4. Line a cookie sheet with a parchment paper or just grease it very well.

5. Drop small balls of about 1 ½ inches wide; then gently flatten the cookies with your hands.

6. Bake your cookies for about 15 minutes; then remove them from the oven and set them aside to cool for about 10 minutes.

7. Serve and enjoy your cookies!

Nutrition Info: Calories: 179;Fat: 17 g;Carbohydrates: 4g;Fiber: 2g;Protein: 5

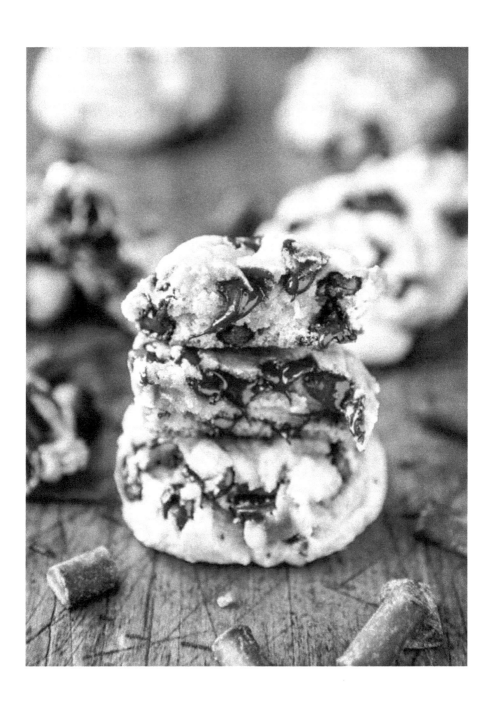

Cream Cheese Cookies

Servings: 24

Cooking Time: 15 Minutes

Ingredients:

- 1 egg white
- 3 cups almond flour
- 1 ½ tsp vanilla
- ½ cup erythritol
- 2 oz cream cheese, softened
- ¼ cup butter softened
- Pinch of salt

Directions:

1. Preheat the oven to 350 F 0 C.
2. Line cookie sheet with parchment paper and set aside.
3. Add butter, sweetener, and cream cheese in food processor and process until fluffy.
4. Add egg white, vanilla, and salt and process well to combine.
5. Add almond flour and process well to combine.
6. Make cookies from mixture and place on prepared cookie sheet.
7. Bake for 15 minutes.
8. Allow to cool completely then serve.

Nutrition Info: Per Servings: Net Carbs: 1.6g; Calories: 107 Total Fat: 7g; Saturated Fat: 2.2g Protein: 3.4g; Carbs: 3.1g; Fiber: 1.5g; Sugar: 0.5g; Fat 82% Protein 13% Carbs 5%

Keto Thumbprint Cookies

Servings: 25-30

Cooking Time: 18 Minutes

Ingredients:

- 2 large eggs, beaten
- 4 cups flour superfine blanched almond flour
- 1 teaspoon baking powder
- 2 teaspoons vanilla extract
- 10 tablespoons sugar-free strawberry preserves
- ¼ cup salted butter, softened
- ¼ teaspoon kosher salt
- 1 1/3 cups powdered erythritol
- 2/3 cup finely chopped walnuts

Directions:

1. Add eggs, flour, baking powder, vanilla, butter, salt and erythritol into a mixing bowl.
2. Mix well into dough.
3. Add walnuts into a shallow bowl.
4. Divide the dough into 25-30 equal portions and shape into balls. Dredge in walnuts.
5. Line 2 large baking sheets with parchment paper.
6. Place the cookies on the baking sheet.
7. Bake in a preheated oven at 350° F for 8 minutes.

8. Remove the baking sheet from the oven. Press each cookie at the center with your thumb to about ½ inch depth.

9. Fill the dents with about a teaspoon of strawberry preserves.

10. Place them back in the oven and bake for minutes.

11. Remove the baking sheet from the oven and let cookies cool completely on the baking sheet.

12. Transfer into an airtight container. These can keep for 5-6 days at room temperature. If you freeze the cookies they can keep for 3 months.

Nutrition Info: per Servings: Calories: .3 kcal, Fat: 12.3 g, Carbohydrates: 4.1 g, Protein: 3.1 g

Keto Chocolate Chip Cookies

Servings: 8

Cooking Time: 16 Minutes

Ingredients:

- 1 cup sunflower seed butter
- 2 eggs
- ¼ cup coconut flour
- 1 tsp vanilla extract
- 1 cup granulated erythritol sweetener
- ¼ cup unsweetened shredded coconut
- 1 tbsp konjac flour
- ¼ tsp kosher salt
- 2 oz coarsely chopped Lindt 90% dark chocolate

Directions:

1. Preheat your oven to 350 degrees F.
2. Mix sunflower seed butter with vanilla, coconut flour, eggs, sweetener, shredded coconut, salt, and konjac flour in a suitably sized bowl.
3. Mix well then fold in chopped chocolate.
4. Make 15 balls out of this mixture then place them on a baking sheet lined with wax paper.
5. Gently press the balls to flatten them into cookies.
6. Bake these cookies for 1minutes until golden brown.
7. Allow them to cool then garnish with salt flakes.

8. Enjoy.

Nutrition Info: Calories 285 Total Fat 17.3 g Saturated Fat 4.5 g Cholesterol 175 mg Sodium 165 mg Total Carbs 3.5 g Sugar 0.4 g Fiber 0.g Protein 7.2 g

Coconut Almond Cookies

Servings: 40

Cooking Time: 10 Minutes

Ingredients:

- 3 cups unsweetened shredded coconut
- 34 cup erythritol
- 1 cup almond flour
- 14 cup can coconut milk

Directions:

1. Spray a baking sheet with cooking spray and set aside.
2. Add all ingredients to a large bowl and mix until combined.
3. Make small balls from mixture and place on a prepared baking sheet and press lightly into a cookie shape.
4. Place in refrigerator until firm.
5. Serve and enjoy.

Nutrition Info: Per Servings: Net Carbs: 0.9g; Calories: 71 Total Fat: 3g; Saturated Fat: 4.4g Protein: 1.2g; Carbs: 2.4g; Fiber: 1.5g; Sugar: 0.7g; Fat 85% Protein 9% Carbs 6%

Butter Pecan

Servings: 10

Cooking Time: 25 Minutes

Ingredients:

- 1/2 cup Swerve sweetener, granulated
- 1/2 tsp. vanilla extract, sugar-free
- 1/2 cup butter, unsalted
- 1 3/4 cups almond flour, blanched
- 1/2 cup pecans, chopped and toasted
- 2 tbsp. coconut flour
- 1/2 tsp. salt

Directions:

1. The stove needs to be set to 325° Fahrenheit. Cover 2 regular sized cookie sheets with baking paper or you can use silicone baking mats instead.
2. Using a big dish, cream the sweetener, vanilla extract, and butter with an electrical beater awaiting the consistency to be fluffy.
3. Combine the almond flour and coconut flour to the mixture until incorporated.
4. Then carefully fold the pecans and salt into the batter.
5. Scoop out the dough with a spoon or cookie scooper. Create 1 inch balls of dough. Lightly press them

approximately 2 inches from each other on the prepared cookie sheets.

6. Heat in the stove for 5 minutes and transfer the cookie sheet to the counter. Use a smooth bottomed glass to press each cookie about 1/4 inches thick.

7. Heat in the stove for another 12 minutes.

8. Leave them to set on the cookie pan for approximately 10 minutes for them to set properly.

Nutrition Info: 3 grams ;Net Carbs: 2.7 grams ;Fat: 11 grams ;Calories: 116

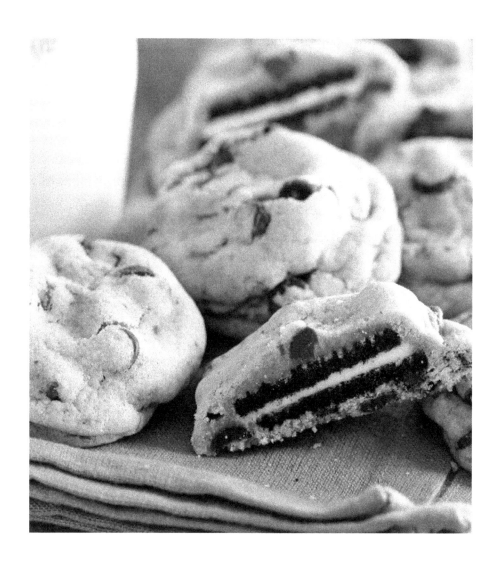

Almond Oreo Cookies

Servings: 25

Cooking Time: 12 Minutes

Ingredients:

- 2 and ¼ cups of hazelnut or almond flour
- 3 Tablespoons of coconut flour
- 4 Tablespoons of cocoa powder
- 1 Teaspoons of baking powder
- ½ Teaspoon of xanthan gum
- ¼ Teaspoon of salt
- ½ Cup of softened butter
- ½ Cup of stevia
- 1 Large egg
- 1 Teaspoon of vanilla extract
- For the Cream Filling:
- 4 Oz of softened cream cheese
- 2 Tablespoons of almond butter
- ½ Teaspoons of pure vanilla extract
- ½ Cup of powdered of Swerve, you can just grind it in a spice grinder

Directions:

1. Preheat your oven to a temperature of about 350 degrees Fahrenheit.

2. Combine the hazelnut or the almond flour with the cocoa powder, the baking powder, the xanthan gum, the salt, the stevia, the egg and the vanilla extract in a large bowl and mix very well.
3. Add the almond butter and mix again.
4. In a separate medium bowl, cream all together the Swerve and the butter until it become light and extremely fluffy for 2 to 3 minutes.
5. Add the egg and the vanilla and mix until your ingredients are fully combined.
6. Add your already mixed dry ingredients and mix it until it is very well combined.
7. Roll out the obtained dough between two rectangular waxed paper sheets; make sure the thickness is about 1/8.
8. Place the dough over a cookie sheet lined with a parchment paper.
9. Roll the cookie dough again until the end.
10. Bake the cookies for about 12 minutes; then let cool completely before starting to fill.
11. To make the filling:
12. Cream the cream cheese with the butter; then cream all together and add the vanilla extract.
13. Gradually add in the powdered swerve.
14. Fill the Oreo cookies with the cream.
15. Serve and enjoy your delicious cookies!

Nutrition Info: Calories: 136;Fat: 12.3 g;Carbohydrates: 2.8g;Fiber: 1.8g;Protein: 4.6 g

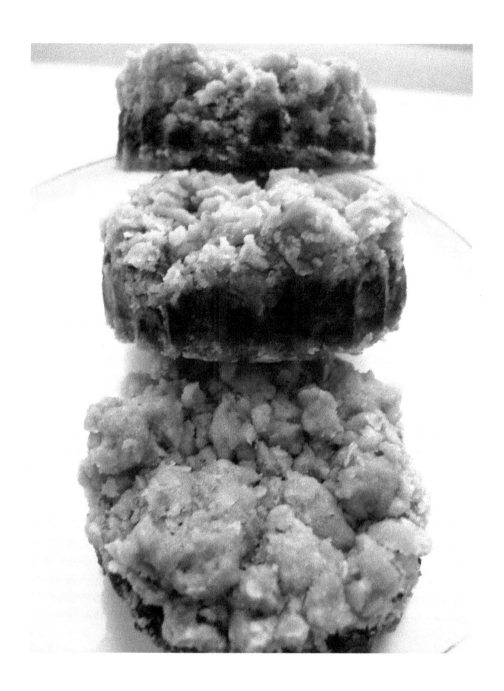

Chocolate Fudge Sandwich Cookies

Servings: 10

Cooking Time:40 Minutes

Ingredients:

- 3 oz 72% cocoa dark chocolate
- 5 oz butter, melted
- 2 eggs
- 3 Tbsp unsweetened cocoa powder
- 1 tsp Stevia/your chosen keto sweetener
- ½ tsp sea salt
- 1 tsp baking powder
- 2 cups ground almonds
- ⅓ cup coconut flour
- Filling:
- 7 oz full fat mascarpone cheese
- ½ tsp Stevia/your chosen keto sweetener
- 1 Tbsp unsweetened cocoa powder

Directions:

1. Preheat the oven to 360 degrees Fahrenheit and line a baking tray with baking paper
2. Place the chocolate and butter into a heatproof bowl over a saucepan of simmering water. Stir as the butter and chocolate melt together, remove from the heat and allow to cool

3. Whisk the eggs, cocoa, stevia and salt into the chocolate mixture

4. Stir the baking powder, ground almonds and cocoa powder into the chocolate/egg mixture until combined

5. Roll the mixture into 20 balls and place them onto your prepared baking tray. Use a fork to press the balls down

6. Pop the tray into the oven and bake for about 15 minutes or until the cookies are just set (they'll still be soft but they'll firm up a little more as they cool)

7. Leave the cookies to cool and make the filling as you wait: simply stir together the mascarpone, sweetener and cocoa powder

8. Spoon a generous dollop of mascarpone filling onto 10 of the cooled cookies and press the other 10 cookies on top so you have 10 sandwich cookies

9. Serve on a platter with a side of hot coffee!

Nutrition Info: Calories: 388;Fat: 36 grams ;Protein: 8 grams ;Total carbs: grams ;Net carbs: 4 grams

Chocolate Dipped Cookies

Servings: 8

Cooking Time: 30 Minutes

Ingredients:

- 1 ½ cups almond flour
- ¼ cup almond butter
- 2 tbsp powdered erythritol
- 1 large egg
- 1 tsp vanilla powder
- 1 tbsp virgin coconut oil
- 1 tbsp coconut butter
- 1 tsp baking powder
- Pinch of salt
- 3.2 oz 90% dark chocolate

Directions:

1. Whisk almond flour, vanilla, salt, baking powder, and erythritol in a mixing bowl.
2. Stir in almond butter, egg, coconut butter, and coconut oil.
3. Mix well to form a dough then place it in a sandwich bag. Refrigerate for minutes.
4. Let your oven preheat at 285 degrees F.
5. Place the dough in between two sheets of parchment then roll it into a ½-inch thick sheet.

6. Use a 2.5-inch diameter cookie cutter to cut the cookies out of this dough.
7. Reroll the remaining dough then place it on a greased baking sheet.
8. Bake the cookies for 30 minutes until golden brown.
9. Place them on a wire rack to cool down.
10. Melt chocolate in a bowl by heating in a microwave and stir well.
11. Dip half of each cooled cookie in the chocolate melt and allow it to set on wax paper.
12. Refrigerate the dipped cookies for 15 minutes.
13. Serve.

Nutrition Info: Calories 236 Total Fat 13.5 g Saturated Fat 4.2 g Cholesterol 541 mg Sodium 21 mg Total Carbs 7.6 g Sugar 1.4 g Fiber 3.8 g Protein 4.3 g

Keto Pumpkin Cheesecake Cookies

Servings: 30

Cooking Time: 20 Minutes

Ingredients:

- For cookies:
- ¾ cup butter, softened
- 2/3 cup solid pack pumpkin puree
- 1 ½ cups granulated erythritol
- 2 teaspoons ground cinnamon
- ¼ teaspoon ground allspice
- ½ teaspoon ground nutmeg
- 4 cups almond flour
- 2 large eggs
- 1 teaspoon baking powder
- ¼ teaspoon salt
- For cheesecake filling:
- 8 ounces cream cheese
- 2 large eggs
- 1 teaspoon vanilla extract
- 4 tablespoons granulated erythritol

Directions:

1. Add butter, pumpkin, sweetener, spices, almond flour, eggs, baking powder and salt into a bowl.
2. Mix with your hands until dough is formed.

3. Scoop mixture into equal portions (about 1 ½ tablespoons dough per cookie) and place on 2 large baking sheets lined with parchment paper.
4. Make a dent on each of the cookies by pressing with the base of the scoop.
5. Add cream cheese, vanilla, eggs and sweetener into a blender and blend until well combined.
6. Spoon the mixture into the dents of the cookies.
7. Bake in a preheated oven at 350° F for about 20 minutes or until golden brown. The cream cheese mixture should have set by now.
8. Remove the baking sheet from the oven and let it cool for – 10 minutes on the baking sheet. Place the cookies on a wire rack to cool completely.
9. Transfer into an airtight container. These can keep for 7 – 8 days in the refrigerator. If you freeze the cookies they can keep for 3 months.

Nutrition Info: per Servings: Calories: 163.1 kcal, Fat: 15.3 g, Carbohydrates: 4 g, Protein: 4.6

Toasted Almond Shortbread Cookies

Servings: 12

Cooking Time: 15 Minutes

Ingredients:

- 2.5 ounces almond flour
- 1/8 teaspoon kosher salt
- 1.5 ounces powdered erythritol
- ¼ teaspoon xanthan gum
- 1.5 ounces butter, at room temperature
- ¼ teaspoon vanilla extract
- For chocolate coating: Optional
- ¼ teaspoon flaky sea salt
- Stevia sweetened chocolate, as required

Directions:

1. Place a skillet over medium heat. When the pan heats, add almond flour and sauté until aromatic and golden brown.
2. Turn off the heat. Add salt and xanthan gum and stir. Let it cool completely.
3. Meanwhile, add butter into a mixing bowl. Beat with an electric mixer for about 2 minutes.
4. Beat in the sweetener. Beat until sweetener dissolves.
5. Beat in the vanilla.

6. Set the mixer on low speed and add about half the almond flour and mix until well combined.

7. Add the remaining flour and mix until well combined.

8. Place the dough on a sheet of cling wrap and wrap the dough. Chill for an hour.

9. Line a baking sheet with parchment paper.

10. Place a sheet of parchment paper or baking paper on your countertop. Place the dough on the center of the sheet. Place another sheet on top of the dough.

11. Roll with a rolling pin until the dough is about ½ inch thick.

12. Use a cookie cutter of about 1 ½ inches diameter and cut the cookies.

13. Place the cookies on the baking sheet. Leave some gap between the cookies.

14. Collect the scrap dough (after cutting into cookies) and reshape into a ball of dough.

15. Repeat steps 10 – 14 (1 – 2 times) and make the remainder of the cookies. Freeze for about minutes.

16. Bake in a preheated oven at 350° F for about 10 – 13 minutes or until light golden brown.

17. Remove the baking sheet from the oven and let the cookies cool on the baking sheet completely.

18. For optional chocolate coating, melt the chocolate in a double boiler. Dip the cookies in chocolate. Sprinkle

flaky sea salt over it. Place in the refrigerator until chocolate sets.

19. Transfer into an airtight container. These can keep for 7 – 8 days in the refrigerator. If you freeze the cookies they can keep for 3 months.

Nutrition Info: per Servings: Calories: 42.1 kcal, Fat: 4.3 g, Carbohydrates: 0.7 g, Protein: 0.7 g

Pistachio Cookies

Servings: 8

Cooking Time: 25 Minutes

Ingredients:

- ¾ cup (4 oz) shelled pistachio nuts
- 2 tsp + 1 cup stevia granulated sweetener
- 1 2/3 cup almond meal or almond flour
- 2 eggs, beaten well

Directions:

1. Add pistachio and stevia to a food processor and pulse until finely ground.
2. Toss pistachio mixture with almond meal or flour in a bowl.
3. Add eggs and whisk well until combined.
4. Refrigerate this mixture for 8 hours or overnight.
5. Let your oven preheat at 32degrees F.
6. Layer a cookie sheet with wax paper then use a scoop or spoon to add the cookie dough to the sheet scoop by scoop.
7. Bake them for 25 minutes until lightly brown.
8. Allow them to cool then serve.

Nutrition Info: Calories 174 Total Fat 12.3 g Saturated Fat 4.8 g Cholesterol 32 mg Sodium 5 mg Total Carbs 4.5 g Fiber 0.6 g Sugar 1.9 g Protein 12 g

Cream Cheese Chocolate Cookies

Servings: 6

Cooking Time: 20 Minutes

Ingredients:

- 1/4 cup of cocoa powder
- 1 cup of coconut flour
- 2 ounces of baking chocolate
- 1 tsp of vanilla essence
- 2 teaspoons of baking powder
- 1/4 teaspoon sea salt
- ½ cup butter, unsalted softened
- 8 ounces cream cheese
- 1 cup swerve
- 1 tsp instant espresso coffee
- 4 eggs
- Chocolate Icing
- A ¼ cup of butter, unsalted
- 1 tsp of MCT oil or coconut oil
- 1/2 cup swerve
- 2-ounce baking chocolate
- ½ tsp instant coffee powder
- Pinch of sea salt

Directions:

1. Cookie Dough

2. Let your oven preheat at 350 degrees F.
3. Melt chocolate in a bowl by heating in the microwave for 20 seconds.
4. Beat cream cheese with vanilla essence, butter, and sweetener in an electric mixer.
5. Continue beating while adding eggs.
6. Add melted chocolate and mix well.
7. Stir in all the dry ingredients and mix again to form a cookie dough.
8. Chocolate Icing
9. Melt butter with chocolate in a bowl by heating in the microwave for 10 seconds.
10. Stir in sweetener, coconut oil, salt, and coffee. Mix well.
11. Baking
12. Divide the cookie dough into flat cookies and place them in a cookie sheet lined with wax paper.
13. Bake them for 20 minutes then allow them to cool.
14. Once cooled, top the cookies with prepared icing.
15. Serve after 5 minutes.

Nutrition Info: Per Servings: Calories 77.88 Total Fat 7.13 g Saturated Fat 4.5 g Cholesterol 15 mg Total Carbs 0.8 g Sugar 0.2 g Fiber 0.3 g Sodium 15 mg Potassium 33 mg Protein 2.3 g

Coconut Lemon Cookies

Servings: 24

Cooking Time: 15 Minutes

Ingredients:

- 4 eggs
- 34 cup Swerve
- 4 oz cream cheese
- 12 cup butter
- 1 12 tsp baking powder
- 1 tbsp lemon peel, grated
- 1 tbsp heavy whipping cream
- 1 tsp lemon extract
- 34 cup coconut flour
- Pinch of salt

Directions:

1. Preheat the oven to 350 F 0 C.
2. Spray a baking tray with cooking spray and set aside.
3. In a bowl, mix together coconut flour, salt, and baking powder. Set aside.
4. In another bowl, add butter, lemon extract, lemon peel, swerve, and cream cheese and beat until well combined.
5. Add eggs one by one and beat until combined.
6. Add whipping cream and stir well to combine.

7. Add coconut flour mixture to the wet mixture and mix until combined.
8. Transfer prepared mixture into the bowl and cover with parchment paper.
9. Place in the refrigerator for 30 minutes.
10. Remove cookie dough from refrigerator and make cookies and place onto a prepared baking tray.
11. Bake for 15 minutes or until lightly brown.
12. Remove from oven and set aside to cool completely.
13. Serve and enjoy.

Nutrition Info: Per Servings: Net Carbs: 0.5g; Calories: 66; Total Fat: 6.5g; Saturated Fat: 3.9g Protein: 1.4g; Carbs: 0.7g; Fiber: 0.2g; Sugar: 0.1g; Fat 89% Protein 9% Carbs 3%

White Chocolate Cranberry Cookies

Servings: 30

Cooking Time: 40 Minutes

Ingredients:
- 1/4 cup dried cranberries, unsweetened
- 3/4 cup coconut flour
- 1 scoop whey protein powder
- 1/16 teaspoon sea salt
- 1/2 cup monk fruit sweetener
- 1/4 cup erythritol sweetener
- 1/2 cup cashew butter

- 1/4 cup white chocolate chips, unsweetened
- Almond milk, as needed

Directions:

1. Place flour in a large bowl, add protein powder, salt, and erythritol and stir until mixed.
2. Add butter and monk fruit sweetener and stir well until the crumbly mixture comes together.
3. Fold in chocolate and berries until incorporated and then slowly mix milk until thick batter comes together.
4. Shape the mixture into small cookie balls, then place them on a cookie sheet lined with parchment paper and press each cookie ball slightly.
5. Place cookie sheet into the refrigerator for 30 minutes or more until firm.
6. Serve straightaway.

Nutrition Info: Calories: 45.5 Cal, Carbs: 1.4g, Fat: 3.6 g, Protein: 1.7 g, Fiber: 1.2 g.

Easy Peanut Butter Cookies

Servings: 15

Cooking Time: 15 Minutes

Ingredients:

- 1 egg
- ½ cup erythritol
- 1 cup peanut butter
- 1 tsp vanilla
- Pinch of salt

Directions:

1. Preheat the oven to 350 F 0 C.
2. Add all ingredients into the large bowl and mix until well combined.
3. Make cookies from bowl mixture and place on a baking tray.
4. Bake in preheated oven for 10-12 minutes.
5. Let it cool completely then serve.

Nutrition Info: Per Servings: Net Carbs: 2.5g; Calories: 10 Total Fat: 8.9g; Saturated Fat: 1.9g Protein: 4.7g; Carbs: 3.5g; Fiber: 1g; Sugar: 1.7g; Fat 75% Protein 17% Carbs 8%

Peanut Butter Muffins

Servings: 12

Cooking Time: 21 Minutes

Ingredients:

- 1 Cup of almond flour
- ½ Cup of So Nourished erythritol
- 1 Teaspoon of baking powder
- 1 Pinch of salt
- 1/3 Cup of peanut butter
- 1/3 Cup of almond milk
- 2 Large eggs
- ½ Cup of cacao nibs

Directions:

1. Preheat your oven to a temperature of about 350 F.
2. In a large mixing bowl; combine the almond flour with the baking powder, the salt and the erythritol.
3. Add the peanut butter and the almond milk and stir.
4. Add in the eggs, one at a time; then stir until each is fully whisked.
5. Add in the cacao nibs and spray a muffin tin with cooking spray.
6. Evenly distribute the batter between the muffin tins and bake for about 20 to 30 minutes.

7. Remove the muffins from the oven and let cool for 5 minutes.

8. Serve and enjoy your delicious muffins!

Nutrition Info: Calories: 265;Fat: 20.4g;Carbohydrates: 4g;Fiber: 2.7g;Protein: 7.6g

Coconut Snowball Cookies

Servings: 40

Cooking Time: 40 Minutes

Ingredients:

- 4 cups shredded coconut, unsweetened
- 1/4 cup monk fruit sweetener
- 1/4 teaspoon vanilla extract, unsweetened
- 1/2 cup coconut milk, unsweetened and full-fat

Directions:

1. Place coconut in a blender and pulse for to 2 minutes at high speed or until fine texture, don't over blend.
2. Add sweetener and milk and continue blending for 1 minute or until thick batter comes together.
3. Tip the mixture into a large bowl and shape into 40 small cookie balls.
4. Place cookie balls on a baking tray lined with parchment paper, and press lightly into a cookie shape.
5. Sprinkle with coconut and place into refrigerator for 30 minutes until firm.
6. Serve straightaway.

Nutrition Info: Calories: 40 Cal, Carbs: 2 g, Fat: 4 g, Protein: 1 g, Fiber: 2 g.

Cheese Chocolate Bars

Servings: 16

Cooking Time: 10 Minutes

Ingredients:

- 16 oz cream cheese, softened
- 14 oz unsweetened dark chocolate
- 1 tsp vanilla
- 12 drops liquid stevia

Directions:

1. Spray 8-inch square pan with cooking spray and set aside.
2. Melt chocolate in a saucepan over low heat.
3. Stir in sweetener and vanilla. Remove from heat and set aside.
4. Add cream cheese into the food processor and process until smooth.
5. Add melted chocolate mixture into the cream cheese and process until well combined.
6. Transfer cheese chocolate mixture into the prepared pan and spread evenly.
7. Place in refrigerator for 4 hours.
8. Slice and serve.

Nutrition Info: Per Servings: Net Carbs: 4.1g; Calories: 265; Total Fat: 23.1g; Saturated Fat: 14.5g Protein: 5.5g;

Carbs: 7.4g; Fiber: 3.3g; Sugar: 0.1g; Fat 82% Protein 11% Carbs 7%

Walnut Coffee Bars

Servings: 12

Cooking Time:45 Minutes

Ingredients:

- 1 cup ground almonds
- 1 cup finely chopped walnuts
- ½ cup ground linseed
- 1 tsp baking powder
- 2 tsp espresso powder dissolved in 1 Tbsp hot water
- 1 tsp Stevia/your preferred keto sweetener
- 2 eggs
- 5 oz butter, melted
- Crumble top:
- 5 oz butter, cold
- 1 cup chopped walnuts
- 1 cup unsweetened coconut thread
- 1 tsp espresso powder
- ½ tsp Stevia/your preferred keto sweetener

Directions:

1. Preheat the oven to 360 degrees Fahrenheit and line a brownie pan with baking paper or grease it thoroughly with butter
2. Combine the ground almonds, walnuts, linseed and baking powder in a large bowl

3. In a separate bowl, whisk together the dissolved espresso, stevia, eggs and butter
4. Pour the wet ingredients into the dry ingredients and stir to thoroughly combine
5. Press the mixture into your prepared pan and set aside as you make the crumble topping
6. Make the crumble topping: using a knife, chop the cooled butter into the walnuts, coconut thread, espresso powder and sweetener until you have a crumbly texture
7. Sprinkle the crumble over top of the base and pop the pan into the oven to bake for about 30 minutes or until golden
8. Leave to cool before slicing and serving!

Nutrition Info: Calories: 422;Fat: 43 grams ;Protein: 8 grams ;Total carbs: 6 grams ;Net carbs: 2 grams

Chocolate Chip Bars

Servings: 24

Cooking Time: 1 Hour

Ingredients:

- 1/3 cup coconut flour
- 1 cup almond flour
- 1 cup chopped walnuts
- 1 1/2 teaspoons baking powder
- 1/2 teaspoon xanthan gum
- 1/4 teaspoon sea salt
- 2 cups swerve sweetener
- 1 cup chocolate chips, stevia sweetened
- 2 teaspoons vanilla extract, unsweetened
- 1/2 cup unsalted butter, softened
- 8-ounce cream cheese, softened
- 5 eggs

Directions:

1. Set oven to 350 degrees F and let preheat.
2. In the meantime, take a 1by 16-inch cookie sheet, line with parchment paper and set aside.
3. Place sweetener, vanilla, butter, and cheese in a bowl and whisk with a stand mixer until smooth.

4. Then beat in eggs, one at a time, until well incorporated and then gently fold in remaining ingredients until combined.

5. Spoon the mixture into prepared cookie sheet, spread evenly and place it into the oven to bake for 30 to 3minutes or until nicely golden brown.

6. When done, let cookie bar cool completely and then slice to serve.

Nutrition Info: Calories: 140 Cal, Carbs: 2.9 g, Fat: 13.5 g, Protein: 4.2 g, Fiber: 0.9 g.

Coconut Bars

Servings: 24

Cooking Time: 10 Minutes

Ingredients:

- ¼ cup of coconut oil
- ½ cup erythritol
- 12 cup coconut cream
- 3 cups unsweetened desiccated coconut

Directions:

1. Line 8*5-inch baking pan with parchment paper and set aside.
2. Add all ingredients into the blender and blend until sticky mixture form.
3. Transfer coconut mixture in prepared baking pan.
4. Spread mixture evenly and press down with your hands.
5. Place in refrigerator for 1minutes.
6. Slice and serve.

Nutrition Info: Per Servings: Net Carbs: 0.2g; Calories: 111; Total Fat: 12g; Saturated Fat: 6g Protein: 0.1g; Carbs: 0.3g; Fiber: 0.1g; Sugar: 0.2g; Fat 98% Protein 1% Carbs 1%

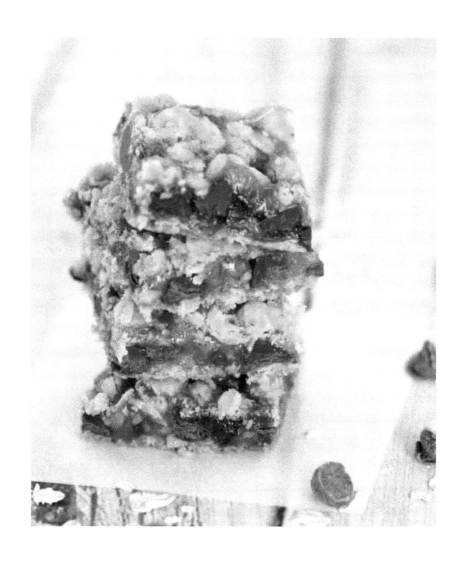

Crunchy Chocolate Bars

Servings: 8

Cooking Time: 0 Minutes

Ingredients:

- 1 1/2 cups sugar-free chocolate chips
- 1 cup almond butter
- Stevia to taste
- 1/4 cup coconut oil
- 3 cups pecans, chopped

Directions:

1. Take an 8-inch baking pan and line it with parchment paper.
2. Melt chocolate chips with sweetener and coconut oil in a glass bowl.
3. Mix well then add seeds and nuts.
4. Pour this nutty batter in the baking pan.
5. Place the pan in the refrigerator for 2 hours.
6. Remove the pan and slice it into
7. Pour this batter into the baking pan and spread evenly.
8. Place it in the refrigerator for 2 hours.
9. Slice in small bars and serve.
10. Enjoy.

Nutrition Info: Calories 316 ;Total Fat 30.9 g ;Saturated Fat 8.1 g ;Cholesterol 0 mg ;Sodium 8 mg ;Total Carbs 8.3 g ;Sugar 1.8 g ;Fiber 3.8 g ;Protein 6.4 g

Saffron Coconut Bars

Servings: 15

Cooking Time: 15 Minutes

Ingredients:

- 1 34 cups unsweetened shredded coconut
- 8 saffron threads
- 1 13 cups unsweetened coconut milk
- 1 tsp cardamom powder
- 14 cup Swerve
- 3.5 oz ghee

Directions:

1. Spray a square baking dish with cooking spray and set aside.
2. In a bowl, mix together coconut milk and shredded coconut and set aside for half an hour.
3. Add sweetener and saffron and mix well to combine.
4. Melt ghee in a pan over medium heat.
5. Add coconut mixture to the pan and cook for 7 minutes.
6. Add cardamom powder and cook for 3-5 minutes more.
7. Transfer coconut mixture into the prepared baking dish and spread evenly.
8. Place in refrigerator for 1-2 hours.

9. Slice and serve.

Nutrition Info: Per Servings: Net Carbs: 1.7g; Calories: 191 Total Fat: 19.2g; Saturated Fat: 15.1g Protein: 1.5g; Carbs: 4.1g; Fiber: 2.4g; Sugar: 1.6g; Fat 91% Protein 5% Carbs 4%

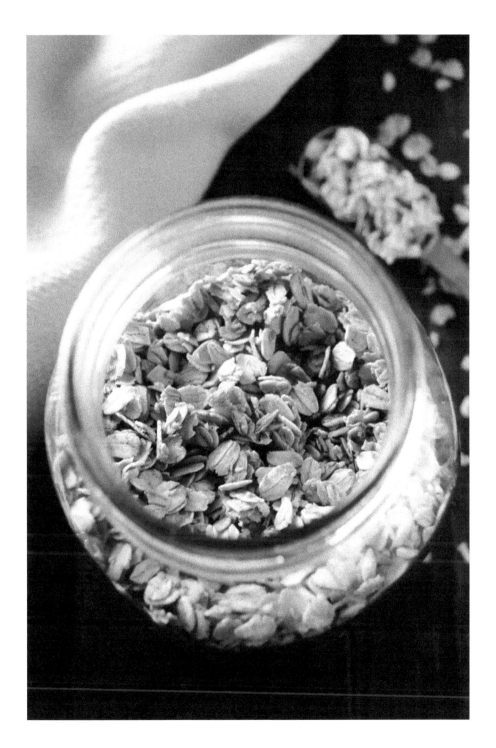

Granola

Servings: 8

Cooking Time: 30 Minutes

Ingredients:

- For the granola:
- 1/3 cup monk fruit sweetener
- 2 tsp. vanilla extract, sugar-free
- 1/4 cup coconut oil
- 1/2 cup almonds, sliced
- 1/4 cup coconut, unsweetened and shredded
- 1/3 cup flaxseed meal
- 1/2 cup almond butter, smooth
- 1/3 cup pumpkin seeds, shelled
- 1 tbsp. chia seeds
- 1/2 tsp. ground cinnamon
- For the drizzle:
- 1 tsp. coconut oil
- 3 tbsp. dark chocolate chips, sugar-free
- For the topping:
- 1 tbsp. almonds, sliced

Directions:

1. Using a regular loaf pan, layer with baking paper and set to the side.

2. Heat a pot to liquefy the sweetener, coconut oil, almond butter, and vanilla extract.

3. In a big dish, combine the almonds and coconut with a rubber scraper. Then add the flaxseed meal, pumpkin seeds, chia seeds, and cinnamon to fully incorporate.

4. Transfer the granola to the prepared pan and press down the mixture by hand to make uniform.Freeze the granola for 20 minutes to harden.In a saucepan, dissolve the chocolate chips and coconut oil together.

5. When set, remove and move the granola onto a serving plate.

6. Dust the almonds on the top and drizzle the chocolate over the almonds. Freeze for 3 additional minutes.

7. Cut into 8 individual bars and enjoy!

8. Tricks and Tips:

9. These granola bars can be individually wrapped in plastic wrap and are perfect for on the go snacks. They will keep for up to 8 days in the refrigerator.

10. Instead of putting the granola in the freezer, you can leave it in the refrigerator overnight to set and complete steps 7 through 9.

Nutrition Info: 8 grams ;Net Carbs: 2.8 grams ;Fat: 28 grams ;Calories: 306

Chocolate Protein Bar

Servings: 8

Cooking Time: 0 Minutes

Ingredients:

- 1 cup nut butter
- 4 tablespoons coconut oil
- 2 scoops vanilla protein
- Stevia, to taste
- ½ teaspoon pink salt
- Optional Ingredients:
- 4 tablespoons sugar-free chocolate chips
- 1 teaspoon cinnamon

Directions:

1. Take a medium-sized dish and mix stevia, with salt, protein, butter and coconut oil.
2. Once well combined, fold in chocolate chop and cinnamon.
3. Spread this mixture into a pan and press it firmly.
4. Refrigerate it for 30 minutes to set it.
5. Slice and serve.

Nutrition Info: Calories 179 ;Total Fat 15.7 g ;Saturated Fat 8 g ;Cholesterol 0 mg ;Sodium 43 mg ;Total Carbs 4.8 g ;Sugar 3.g ;Fiber 0.8 g ;Protein 5.6 g

Cocoa Bars

Servings: 12

Cooking Time: 5-7 Minutes

Ingredients:

- 0.7 ounce raw cacao butter
- 1 teaspoon maca powder
- 1 tablespoon unsweetened cocoa powder
- 1 tablespoon 100% CB liquid MCT oil
- 1/8 teaspoon ground cinnamon (optional)

Directions:

1. Add cacao butter, maca powder, cocoa powder oil and cinnamon into a small pot.
2. Place the pot over low heat. Stir frequently until the cacao butter melts.
3. Remove from heat and whisk until well combined.
4. Spoon into chocolate bar silicone molds and cool completely.
5. Place in the freezer and freeze until firm.
6. Remove from the molds and serve.
7. Leftovers can be stored in an airtight container in the refrigerator. These can keep for 4 – 5 days.

Nutrition Info: Per Servings: Calories: 23.6 kcal, Fat: 2.g, Carbohydrates: 0.4 g, Protein: 0.2 g

Blueberry Bars

Servings: 4

Cooking Time: 75 Minutes

Ingredients:

- ¼ cup blueberries
- 1 tsp vanilla
- 1 tsp fresh lemon juice
- 2 tbsp erythritol
- ¼ cup almonds, sliced
- ¼ cup coconut flakes
- 3 tbsp coconut oil
- 2 tbsp coconut flour
- ½ cup almond flour
- 3 tbsp water
- 1 tbsp chia seeds

Directions:

1. Preheat the oven to 300 F 0 C.
2. Line baking dish with parchment paper and set aside.
3. In a small bowl, mix together water and chia seeds. Set aside.
4. In a bowl, combine together all ingredients. Add chia mixture and stir well.
5. Pour mixture into the prepared baking dish and spread evenly.

6. Bake for 50 minutes. Remove from oven and allow to cool completely.

7. Cut into bars and serve.

Nutrition Info: Per Servings: Net Carbs: 2.; Calories: 136; Total Fat: 11.9g; Saturated Fat: 6.1g Protein: 3.1g; Carbs: 5.5g; Fiber: 2.7g; Sugar: 1.3g; Fat 81% Protein 10% Carbs 9%

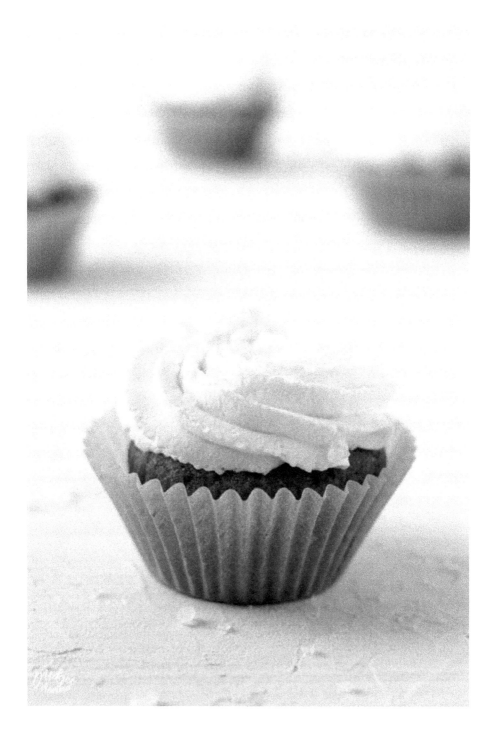

Low-carb Coconut Macadamia Bars

Servings: 32

Cooking Time: 55-60 Minutes

Ingredients:

- For crust:
- 2 ½ cups almond flour
- ½ teaspoon salt
- 2/3 cup Swerve sweetener
- 8 tablespoons unsalted butter, chilled, cut into small cubes
- For filling:
- ½ cup butter
- 1 cup coconut cream
- 1 ½ cups chopped macadamia nuts
- 1 teaspoon vanilla extract
- 1 cup Swerve sweetener
- 2 2/3 cups flaked coconut
- 2 egg yolks

Directions:

1. To make crust: Add almond flour, salt and sweetener into the food processor bowl. Process until well incorporated.
2. Scatter the butter cubes and pulse until crumbly.
3. Line a large baking (19) dish with parchment paper.

4. Transfer the mixture into the baking dish. Press well on the bottom of the dish.

5. Bake in a preheated oven at 3° F for about 20-25 minutes or until light brown. Remove from the oven and set aside to cool for a while.

6. Meanwhile, make the filling as follows: Add butter into a saucepan. Place over medium heat.

7. When butter melts, add sweetener and coconut cream and whisk until well combined.

8. Add nuts, coconut, vanilla and yolks and whisk until well incorporated. Turn off the heat.

9. Spread the mixture over the crust.

10. Bake until golden brown on the edges. The center may look slightly undercooked but that's ok, it will harden when it cools. Cool completely.

11. Cut into 32 bars and serve.

12. Leftovers can be stored in an airtight container in the refrigerator. These can keep for 4 – 5 days.

Nutrition Info: Per Servings: Calories: 198.7 kcal, Fat: 15.7 g, Carbohydrates: 5.9 g, Protein: 3 g

Sukrin Protein Bars

Servings: 8

Cooking Time: 2 Minutes

Ingredients:

- 2 oz. butter
- 6 oz. Sukrin Gold Fibber Syrup
- 3 oz. thickened cream
- 3 oz. whey protein powder
- 0.4 oz. Sukrin Melis
- 1 teaspoon vanilla essence
- 1 pinch sea salt flakes
- Nougat Layer
- 3 oz. Sukrin Clear Fibber Syrup
- 2 oz. whey protein isolate
- 0.4 oz. cacao powder

Directions:

1. Caramel Layer
2. Cook all of its ingredients in a suitable glass bowl in the microwave for minutes.
3. Once melted, mix well then divide the mixture into two glass bowls.
4. Heat the one half for 1 minute more in the microwave to thicken it.

5. Mix the other half with sukrin, salt, vanilla, and protein.

6. Divide it into molds of a tray.

7. Top each of the molds with thickened caramel sauce.

8. Chocolate Layer

9. To prepare this layer, cook fiber syrup for 2 minutes in the microwave.

10. Then add protein and cacao powder to it.

11. Mix well well then pour it over the caramel layer in each mold.

12. Refrigerate it for 30 minutes or more.

13. Serve and enjoy.

Nutrition Info: Calories 331 ;Total Fat 32.9 g ;Saturated Fat 6.1 g ;Cholesterol 10 mg ;Sodium 18 mg ;Total Carbs 9.1 g ;Sugar 2.8 g ;Fiber 0.8 g ;Protein 4.4 g

Lime Mixed Shortbread Bars

Servings: 8

Cooking Time: 35 Minutes

Ingredients:
- Shortbread Crust:
- 1 1/4 cups almond flour
- 1/3 cup Swerve
- 1/4 teaspoon salt
- 1/4 cup butter melted

Directions:
1. Crust:
2. Let your oven preheat at 3 degrees F.
3. Combine sweetener with salt and almond flour in a suitable bowl.
4. Add in melted butter and then pour it in an 8inch pan.
5. Press the crust firmly and then bake it for 1minutes in the preheated oven.
6. Once done, allow it to cool at room temperature for 15 minutes.
7. Lime Filling:
8. Beat the cream cheese with egg yolks and lime zest during this time.
9. Once smooth and foamy, whisk in lime juice and milk in the mixture.

10. Spread this filling in the baked crust and return the pan to the oven for 20 minutes.

11. Once done, allow it to cool for 10 minutes at room temperature.

12. Slice the base into bars then garnish as desired.

13. Enjoy.

Nutrition Info: Calories 220 ;Total Fat 20.1 g ;Saturated Fat 7.4 g ;Cholesterol 132 mg ;Sodium 157 mg ;Total Carbs 63 g ;Sugar 0.4 g ;Fiber 2.4 g ;Protein 6.1 g

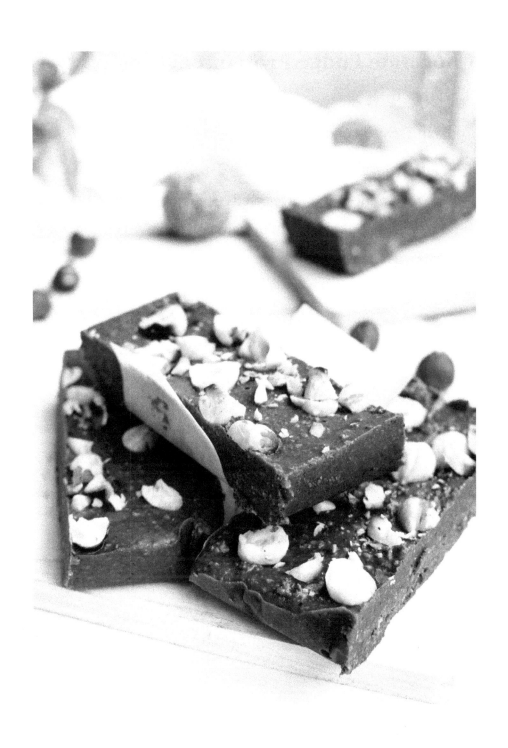

Chocolate Fudge Protein Bars

Servings: 16

Cooking Time: 1 Hour And 10 Minutes

Ingredients:

- 4 ounces sunflower seeds
- 2 scoops chocolate protein powder
- 1/2 teaspoon salt
- 3/4 cup swerve sweetener
- 3 ounces cocoa powder, unsweetened
- 8 tablespoons coconut oil
- 4 ounces tahini

Directions:

1. Place all the ingredients in a blender or food processor and pulse for 2 to 3 minutes or until smooth, scraping the sides of the container.
2. Take a loaf pan, line with parchment paper, then spoon in prepared batter and spread evenly.
3. Place loaf pan into the refrigerator and refrigerate for minutes or until firm.
4. Then cut into 8 bars and cut each bar to make 16 bars.
5. Continue freezing for 30 minutes or until hard and then serve.

Nutrition Info: Calories: 159 Cal, Carbs: 3.g, Fat: 14.8 g, Protein: 6.7 g, Fiber: 1.5 g.

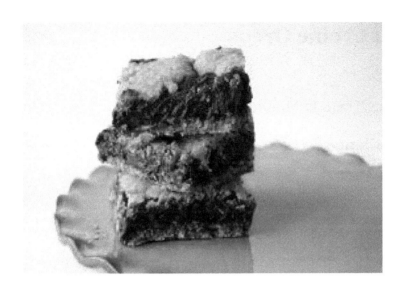

Mint Creme Oreos

Servings: 12

Cooking Time: 12 Minutes

Ingredients:

- 2 ¼ cups almond flour
- 3 tbsp coconut flour
- 4 tbsp cacao powder
- 1 tsp baking powder
- 1 ½ tsp xanthan gum
- ¼ tsp salt
- ½ cup grass-fed butter, unsalted and softened
- 1 egg
- 1 tsp vanilla extract
- 4 oz cream cheese
- 1 cup lakanto monk fruit
- 1 tsp peppermint extract

Directions:

1. Preheat your oven to 350 degrees F.
2. Mix coconut flour with almond flour, xanthan gum, salt, baking powder, and cocoa powder in a medium-sized bowl.
3. Whisk ½ cup monk fruit sweetener with six tablespoons of butter in a bowl until fluffy.

4. Add vanilla extract and egg then beat well and stir in dry ingredients to form the dough.
5. Place this dough in between two sheets of wax paper and roll it into a 1/8-inch thick sheet.
6. Cut cookies with a round cookie cutter then re-roll the remaining dough to cut more cookies.
7. Place these cookies on a cookie sheet lined with parchment paper.
8. Bake these cookies for 12 minutes then allow them to cool.
9. Meanwhile, beat cream cheese with 2 tablespoons butter, ½ cup monk fruit, and peppermint extract in a small bowl.
10. Divide this mixture over half of the cookies.
11. Place the remaining half of the cookies over the cream filling.
12. Press the two halves together gently.
13. Enjoy.

Nutrition Info: Calories 331 Total Fat 12.9 g Saturated Fat 6.1 g Cholesterol 10 mg Sodium 18 mg Total Carbs 9.1 g Sugar 2.8 g Fiber 0.8 g Protein 4.4 g

Keto Oreos

Servings: 6

Cooking Time: 12 Minutes

Ingredients:
- Cookies
- 1/4 teaspoon salt
- 4 tablespoons cocoa powder
- 1 egg
- 3 tablespoons coconut flour
- 2 1/4 cups almond flour
- 1/2 teaspoon xanthan gum
- 1/2 cup swerve
- 1 teaspoons baking powder
- 1/2 cup butter, softened
- 1 teaspoon vanilla essence
- Filling
- 2 tablespoons butter
- 4 oz. cream cheese, softened
- 1/2 teaspoons vanilla essence
- 1/2 cup powdered Swerve

Directions:
1. Let your oven preheat at 350 degrees F.
2. Toss all the dry ingredients in a suitably sized bowl.

3. Beat cream with swerve and butter in an electric mixer until fluffy for 2 minutes.
4. Add vanilla and egg while mixing the mixture.
5. Stir in dry ingredients and mix thoroughly.
6. Spread this dough into 1/8-inch-thick sheet between two wax paper.
7. Cut the dough into cookies using a cookie cutter.
8. Place the cookies in the baking sheet lined with wax paper.
9. Bake them for 12 minutes then allow them to cool.
10. To make the filling
11. Meanwhile, beat cream with butter, vanilla and cream cheese in a mixer.
12. Spread the cream filling on top of half of the biscuits.
13. Place the remaining biscuits over the filling.
14. Serve.

Nutrition Info: Per Servings: Calories 114 Total Fat 9.6 g Saturated Fat 4.5 g Cholesterol 10 mg Total Carbs 3.1 g Sugar 1.4 g Fiber 1.5 g Sodium mg Potassium 93 mg Protein 3.5 g

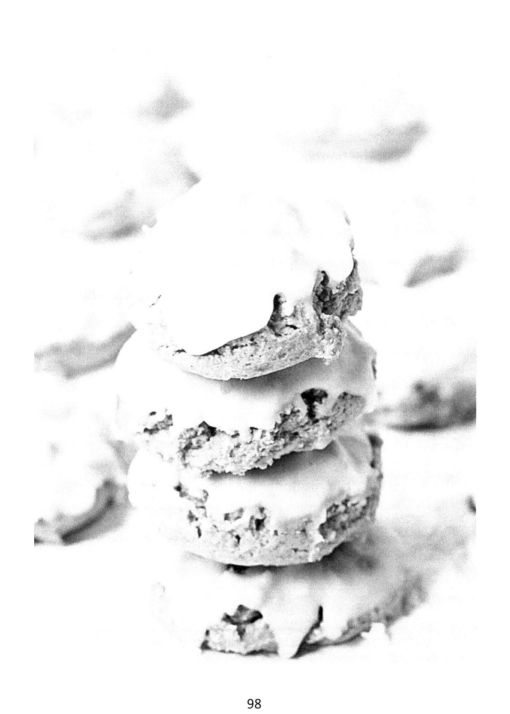

Vanilla Cream Cheese Cookies

Servings: 8

Cooking Time: 15 Minutes

Ingredients:

- 1/4 cup butter
- 2 oz. plain cream cheese
- 1/2 cup erythritol
- 1 large egg white
- 2 teaspoons vanilla essence
- 3 cup almond flour
- 1/4 teaspoon sea salt

Directions:

1. Let your oven preheat at 350 degrees F.
2. Line a cookie sheet with wax paper.
3. Blend butter, cream cheese, egg white and vanilla essence in a blender.
4. Add flour, erythritol, and salt, and mix well until smooth.
5. Divide the dough into small cookies on the cookie sheet.
6. Bake for 15 mins in the preheated oven.
7. Allow the cookies to cool in 15 minutes.
8. Serve.

Nutrition Info: Calories 1 ;Total Fat 14.3 g ;Saturated Fat 10.5 g ;Cholesterol 175 mg ;Sodium 125 mg ;Total Carbs 4.5 g ;Sugar 0.5 g ;Fiber 0.3 g ;Protein 3.2 g

Simple Chocolate Cookies

Servings: 20

Cooking Time: 10 Minutes

Ingredients:

- 3 tbsp ground chia
- 1 cup almond flour
- 2 tbsp chocolate protein powder
- 1 cup sunflower seed butter

Directions:

1. Preheat the oven to 350 F 0 C.
2. Spray a baking sheet with cooking spray and set aside.
3. In a large bowl, add all ingredients and mix until combined.
4. Make small balls from mixture and place on a prepared baking sheet.
5. Press lightly into a cookie shape.
6. Bake in for 10 minutes.
7. Allow to cool completely then serve.

Nutrition Info: Per Servings: Net Carbs: 4.2g; Calories: 111; Total Fat: 9.3g; Saturated Fat: 0.9g Protein: 4g; Carbs: 5.2g; Fiber: 1g; Sugar: 0.2g; Fat 73% Protein 13% Carbs 14%

Coconut Cookies

Servings: 40

Cooking Time: 40 Minutes

Ingredients:

- 1 cup chocolate chips, unsweetened
- 1 cup almond flour
- 3 cups shredded coconut, unsweetened
- 3/4 cup monk fruit sweetener
- 1/4 cup coconut milk, unsweetened and full-fat

Directions:

1. Place all the ingredients in a blender and pulse at high speed for to 2 minutes or until incorporated and thick batter comes together.
2. Shape mixture into 40 cookie balls and place on a large baking tray, lined with parchment paper.
3. Place the baking tray into the refrigerator for minutes until cookies are firm. Serve straightaway.

Nutrition Info: Calories: Cal, Carbs: 2 g, Fat: 4 g, Protein: 1 g, Fiber: 2 g.

Brownie Cookies

Servings: 14

Cooking Time: 10 Minutes

Ingredients:

- 1 egg
- 3 tbsp unsweetened almond milk
- ¼ cup unsweetened chocolate chips
- ½ cup erythritol
- ¼ cup unsweetened cocoa powder
- 1 cup almond butter

Directions:

1. Preheat the oven to 350 F 0 C.
2. Line baking tray with parchment paper and set aside.
3. In a bowl, mix together almond butter, egg, sweetener, almond milk, and cocoa powder until well combined.
4. Stir in Chocó chips.
5. Make cookies from mixture and place on a prepared baking tray.
6. Bake for 10 minutes.
7. Allow to cool completely then serve.

Nutrition Info: Per Servings: Net Carbs: 1g; Calories: 44; Total Fat: 3.5g; Saturated Fat: 1.7g Protein: 1.5g; Carbs: 2.2g; Fiber: 1.2g; Sugar: 0.1g; Fat 75% Protein 15% Carbs 10%

Hazelnut Flour Cookies

Servings: 6

Cooking Time: 25 Minutes

Ingredients:

- 1 cup hazelnut meal ground
- 2 egg whites
- 1 tbsp powdered erythritol
- 10 drops vanilla stevia glycerite
- 1 tsp vanilla
- crushed hazelnuts to decorate

Directions:

1. Swiftly beat egg whites in an electric mixer until they form peaks.
2. Gently fold in hazelnut meal, vanilla, stevia, and erythritol.
3. Mix well then drop the dough scoop by scoop over a baking sheet lined with parchment paper.
4. Flatten each scoop into flat cookies and bake them for 25 minutes at 320 degrees F.
5. Allow them to cool then serve.
6. Enjoy.

Nutrition Info: Per Servings: Calories 151 Total Fat 14.g Saturated Fat 1.5 g Cholesterol 13 mg Total Carbs 1.5 g Sugar

0.3 g Fiber 0.1 g Sodium 53 mg Potassium 131 mg Protein 0.8 g

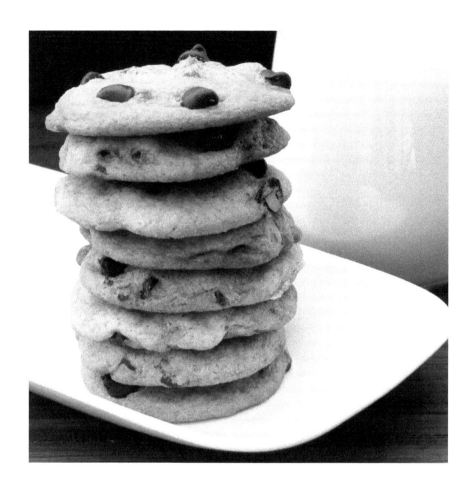

Chocolate Chip Butter Cookies

Servings: 8

Cooking Time: 15 Minutes

Ingredients:

- ¼ cup coconut flour
- ⅓ cup butter, unsalted
- 3 tablespoons Swerve
- 2 eggs, large
- 3 tablespoons sugar-free chocolate chips
- ¼ teaspoon vanilla essence
- ⅛ teaspoon salt

Directions:

1. Mix salt, swerve and coconut flour in a suitable bowl.
2. Beat the vanilla essence and butter in egg in a mixer.
3. Stir in the sweetened flour mixture and mix well to combine.
4. Fold in chocolate chips then drop this batter spoon by spoon on a cookie sheet.
5. Make as many cookies to use the complete batter.
6. Bake the set cookies in the preheated oven for 15 mins at 350 degrees F.
7. Let them cool first then serve.

Nutrition Info: Calories 19;Total Fat 19.2 g ;Saturated Fat 11.5 g ;Cholesterol 123 mg ;Sodium 142 mg ;Total Carbs 4.5 g ;Sugar 3.3 g ;Fiber 0.3 g ;Protein 3.4 g

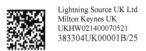
Lightning Source UK Ltd.
Milton Keynes UK
UKHW021400070521
383304UK00001B/25